THE ABELLA MODEL

Leading High-Stress Professionals with Trauma-Informed Practices

————

Lita E. Abella
JD, BCC, ACC

The ABELLA Model: Leading High-Stress Professionals with Trauma-Informed Practices

By: Lita E. Abella, JD, BCC, ACC

ISBN Audiobook: 979-8-9996611-2-8

ISBN Print book: 979-8-9996611-1-1

ISBN eBook: 979-8-9996611-0-4

Cover design: Lita Abella

Published by: Abella & Associates Group LLC

Printed in the United States

First Edition 2025

NOTICE: The information contained in this book is provided for informational and educational purposes only. It is not intended as, and should not be interpreted as, legal, medical, or professional advice. The content is based on the author's years of experience, education, training, research, and review of relevant literature, as well as insights gathered from interviews and discussions with subject matter experts and other professionals in related fields.

Every individual's circumstances are unique, and the strategies, frameworks, and recommendations discussed in this book may not be suitable for everyone. Readers are encouraged to consult with qualified healthcare providers, legal professionals, or other experts regarding their specific needs before making decisions or implementing any practices described herein.

The author and publisher expressly disclaim any liability for adverse effects arising directly or indirectly from the use or application of the information in this book. By reading this book, you acknowledge and agree that you are responsible for your own choices and actions.

To those who carry the weight of others' pain and keep going—

To the legal, healthcare, public service, and other dedicated professionals who show up for others, even when the cost is invisible.

You are not broken. You are brave.

This book is for you—may it offer the validation you've longed for, the healing you deserve, and the recognition you've earned.

It is a tribute to your resilience, your sacrifice, and your humanity.

To my brother, his family, my sister, and my extended family, I love you all from the bottom of my heart.

And to my son, Christian—the person I love most in this world.

Watching you grow into the man, the advocate, and the attorney you are today fills me with more pride than words can hold. Being your mom has been the hardest job I've ever had—and the most beautiful, meaningful, and rewarding one. You are my heart, my inspiration, and my greatest joy.

With all my love,
Lita E. Abella

ADVANCE PRAISE FOR
THE ABELLA MODEL

"The ABELLA Model *presents a framework for individuals in high-stress professions, equipping them with essential trauma-informed practices. This book is both candid and brave, featuring Ms. Abella's personal experiences while providing invaluable guidance for prioritizing well-being. This is a great resource for lawyers and others in the legal profession.*"

~Jennifer Johnston Terando, R.N., Esq.

"*Lita bravely reveals how her own intense personal and professional experiences significantly impacted her mental health, sparking her passion to guide other professionals through similar challenges.* The ABELLA Model *offers a profound exploration of the physiological toll that high-pressure careers, compounded by personal adversities, can take on an individual. Through this framework, Lita equips readers with tangible strategies they can implement to regain control of their lives and mental health.*"

~Jasmin E. Darron, Esq.

"Whether someone is navigating their own challenges or leading teams through crisis and complexity, this book provides practical tools and fresh perspectives to help them thrive. I highly recommend The ABELLA Model *to legal professionals, firm leaders, and anyone committed to cultivating resilience in the workplace."*

~Melinda Gagyor, Legal Recruiter

"If you're a professional, work within an organization, or are self-employed, this very personal, inspirational narrative is a must-read. Whether you feel overwhelmed, stressed, or simply stuck in your routine, this book will open your eyes to the many ways trauma can impact you and those around you."

~Carol Arias, Retired Educator of 40 years

"Filled with useful examples from the school of life, this slim volume offers a wealth of insights into the dynamics of personal change. If you want to bring meaningful change to a stress-filled life, read this book and follow each of the steps it details."

~Bruce Monroe, Retired Government Attorney

"Lita Abella has created a valuable tool designed specifically for high-stress professions. In The ABELLA Model, *readers will find heart, solutions, power, assistance, and support to recraft their own futures and avoid the inevitable breaking points of severe trauma unaddressed. I recommend this book and the help it offers to individuals, teams, departments, and organizations."*

~Susan Zytnik-Künzler, MSOL, ACC, BCC, CBC, Credentialed Coach

"Lita's recovery from a traumatic time and her development of The ABELLA Model *for assessing and addressing well-being are based on real-life experiences of trauma transformed into a pathway for the*

sustainable practice of well-being. A must-read for all individuals and institutions, and especially for those in law enforcement, government oversight, and emergency services."

~Caroline Vincent, Attorney and Mediator

TABLE OF CONTENTS

BEFORE WE BEGIN...

Dear Reader,

Thank you for joining me on this journey—one that I know, from both my own experience and my work with countless professionals, can be both challenging and deeply rewarding. I wrote this book because I understand, firsthand, how difficult it can be to face substance use, mental health struggles, and the invisible wounds of trauma, especially in the high-stakes environments we serve. I've been there myself, and I've walked alongside others who have felt isolated, misunderstood, or simply exhausted by the weight of their responsibilities.

The ABELLA Model™ you'll discover here is more than a framework—it's a lifeline. Born from my years in law enforcement and as a coach, consultant, and legal professional—then refined through my own healing journey with the guidance of therapists, coaches, and mental health experts—this model offers a clear, actionable path out of denial and coping (which can get messy) and moves you (or your entire organization) toward true resilience. Each chapter is designed to feel like a conversation with a trusted mentor, packed with insights, real-world strategies, and moments of recognition that will make you pause, reflect, and take the next step forward.

But this book is just the beginning. I invite you to visit my website, **www.LitaAbella.com**, and take my *free self-assessment*. In just a few minutes, you'll gain eye-opening clarity about how trauma may be affecting you, both personally and professionally. I hope that, as you read, you'll not only find yourself unable to put this book down, but also inspired to take action. Together, let's move from (barely) surviving to (sustainably) thriving.

Stay safe, strong, fit, and healthy—and remember, you are not alone. The journey starts now. I am here when you want to connect: Lita@LitaAbella.com.

Warmly,
Lita E. Abella, JD

IT WAS ALMOST MY LAST CALL

It wasn't until I was arrested for a DUI in 2009 that I finally stopped drinking to cope with the demands of my job and its impact on my life.

That night, I was feeling sorry for myself. All I seemed to do was work, work, work—and I felt that I *deserved* a night out. So I got all dressed up and drove to a nightclub in Orange County. I was extremely depressed, exhausted, and I drank more than I should have. Soon, it was late, and the club was closing. I knew I should not drive—but I got into my car anyway. I had to drive at least 30 miles to get home.

I entered the freeway via the exit ramp, the wrong way. I only realized it when I saw other cars coming towards me. Thank God, I was alert enough to back up and exit the freeway. I finally was able to find the proper entrance to the freeway, and I prayed that I would make it home safely without killing myself or anyone else.

I was one off-ramp from my exit on the freeway when I saw lights behind me. I immediately exited the freeway and pulled over. The California Highway Patrol officers exited their vehicle. I knew I was in trouble. After asking me the usual questions and conducting the Field Sobriety Test on me—which I failed—I was arrested for Driving Under the Influence, Section 23152 of the California Vehicle Code. A code I knew very well, because I had arrested hundreds of motorists for the same offense myself.

Growing up with an abusive mother, moving on to an abusive husband, into a dangerous, but exciting career, married and divorced twice to another abusive husband, then graduating from law school, and starting a business—all while raising a child as a single mom, and taking care of my then-ailing mother—was *indeed* very stressful.

I had adapted to a certain level of stress that really wasn't healthy, because I was surrounded by it. That had become my "normal," and my reference point. I told myself I didn't have time to unwind any other way or take proper care of myself. *Look at all the things I was doing.* I believe that the DUI arrest saved my life. The awful experience I endured being pulled over, handcuffed, and taken to the station, however, is something I never want to experience again in my life.

Luckily, since I had no prior arrest records, I was only cited and released. The few hours that I was in a holding cell, however, were extremely traumatic. Ordinarily, I was the person who would put an arrestee in the holding cell. It was a physically, emotionally, and mentally traumatic and humiliating experience, not to mention *incredibly* expensive. I had to hire an attorney to represent me in my criminal matter and my DMV hearing, and that cost a lot of money, along with the hours I had to put in to attend the alcohol education classes. This added up to an awful lot of time taken away from work and from my son.

The arrest was the "slap in my face" that I needed to stop self-medicating with alcohol and seek other ways of dealing with the trauma, stress, anxiety, and depression I suffered from during those years.

It started me on a journey of understanding what was beneath my unsolvable problems, stubborn stress, and the culture all around me, where people who were "helpers" never asked for any help with processing the horrific things they experienced on the job, despite accumulating traumatic exposure like a snowball down a mountain. Faster, bigger, and more, until it was unstoppable and terrifying.

Should you fail to recognize the early warning signs of mental health issues such as PTSD, vicarious trauma, compassion fatigue, and burnout, then the potential for significant physical, mental, and emotional decline increases.

Knowing sound strategies in dealing with these issues is crucial for your effective coping and recovery.

This is not solely a problem at the individual level, make no mistake. *If your organization fails to cultivate a deeply trauma- informed culture and instead treats cumulative trauma as "just part of the job," then you risk compounding harm, diminishing the effectiveness and well-being of your professionals, increasing liability and staff turnover, and ultimately undermining your mission to serve with true empathy and effectiveness.*

First, let me provide a brief high-level overview of what PTSD, vicarious trauma, compassion fatigue, and burnout are.

Post-Traumatic Stress Disorder (PTSD)

According to the US Department of Veterans Affairs, about 6 out of every 100 people (or 6% of the U.S. population) will have PTSD at some point in their lives.[1] The National Library of Medicine states, "PTSD is particularly prevalent among certain occupational groups, such as police officers, firefighters, medical workers, and military personnel, all of whom can experience events that might trigger PTSD."[2]

The Diagnostic and Statistical Manual of Mental Disorders, Fifth Edition (DSM-5), defines Post-Traumatic Stress Disorder as the result of exposure to a traumatic event (directly experiencing, witnessing, or learning about it), leading to symptoms lasting more than one month, including intrusive memories, avoidance, negative mood changes, and hyperarousal.

In other words, it is a traumatic event that occurred to you, a close family member, or friend, or you witnessed it.

Vicarious Trauma

According to the Substance Abuse and Mental Health Services Administration, 90% of patients/clients seen in public healthcare settings have experienced trauma, and between 40% and 80%

1   National Center for PTSD. 2023. "How Common Is PTSD in Adults?" U.S. Department of Veteran Affairs. February 3, 2023.

2   Coenen, Pieter, and Henk F van der Molen. 2021. "What Work- Related Exposures Are Associated with Post-Traumatic Stress Disorder? A Systematic Review with Meta-Analysis." BMJ Open 11 (8): e049651. https://doi.org/10.1136/bmjopen-2021-049651.

of helping professionals develop vicarious trauma, compassion fatigue, and/or traumatic symptoms.

The American Counseling Association defines Vicarious Trauma as the emotional residue of exposure to traumatic stories and experiences of others through work; witnessing fear, pain, and terror that others have experienced; a preoccupation with horrific stories told to the professional. It is also known as secondary traumatic stress. It is not a diagnosis itself, but its symptoms can be criteria for PTSD.

Vicarious trauma is different from PTSD because it is usually from repeated stories and experiences of *others* told to you, mainly as part of one's job (therapist, police officer, counselor, attorney, journalist, public servant, etc.).

Compassion Fatigue

The American Psychological Association (APA) defines Compassion Fatigue as the physical, emotional, and psychological distress experienced by those who work in helping professions, stemming from repeated exposure to trauma or suffering in others. It's often described as a "cost of caring" and can manifest as exhaustion, withdrawal, and a diminished capacity for empathy.

Compassion fatigue is recognized as an occupational hazard for professionals who frequently engage with individuals experiencing emotional or physical pain. It is not a specific mental health diagnosis but a concept used in therapy and outreach.

Burnout

The American Psychological Association (APA) states, "a significant number of workers experience burnout, with some surveys indicating that over half of the workforce is affected."

The APA defines burnout as a psychological syndrome characterized by emotional exhaustion, cynicism, and reduced professional efficacy resulting from prolonged exposure to chronic workplace stress. It's a state where individuals feel drained, detached from their work, and ineffective in their roles. While burnout is recognized by the World Health Organization (WHO) as an "occupational phenomenon," it is not considered a mental disorder or medical diagnosis.

Compassion fatigue and burnout, while sharing some similarities, are distinct concepts. Compassion fatigue is a form of secondary traumatic stress from helping others, whereas burnout is a more general exhaustion and disengagement from one's work.

Compassion fatigue, vicarious trauma, and burnout can also be experienced simultaneously, as these conditions often interact and exacerbate each other due to the intense emotional demands of their work. Very often, if a client presents with "unsolvable" problems, I find that they have more than one layer of occupational (or otherwise) impairment in this area. If only one is addressed, a reasonable likelihood exists that the person will not respond fully to the protocols for that issue, and unpacking the other conditions will be necessary.

Understanding the realities of PTSD, vicarious trauma, compassion fatigue, and burnout is only the beginning. While these definitions help us recognize the challenges we face, they also underscore the urgent need for practical, compassionate solutions.

Uncovering the Origins of Your Trauma

I created The ABELLA Model to help guide you through a clear, actionable process to uncover the traumatic origins of stubborn problems professionals like you tend to have, whether you know it's about trauma or not. We start from recognizing and confronting the most common patterns we fall into in response, which are avoidance and blame. Once we have a handle on the role those have played in our lives to this point, we can begin evaluating how trauma-related issues have personally impacted you, what you can do about it starting now, and learn what it really means to take personal responsibility and heal.

I say personal responsibility here, but many of my clients are actually leaders or employee assistance personnel in organizations where trauma, compassion fatigue, burnout, and similar issues have eroded a culture or made it difficult to engage, retain, and preserve the well-being of dedicated employees. Those clients grasp that at an organizational level, as well as for individuals within it, there is a human cost to the chronic exposure to events, subject matter, and emotions that needs to be addressed, or else it can turn into unsolved and unsolvable problems.

Healing is possible with guidance and a commitment to some deep emotional work, yet until we can understand that the root of what feels beyond our ability to cope is the trauma we carry, we will continue to avoid, blame, and shrink from the rest of our lives.

My framework is different because many frameworks available focus either on organizational policies or individual self-care, but rarely bridge both. My framework works differently: It acknowledges the "why now" factor, creates a point of choice for the individual or organization to change their way of thinking and behaving around trauma, leverages existing support systems, validates without victimizing, and is scalable to whole organizations.

Staying comfortable or silent in the face of these challenges may offer short-term relief, but over time, it increases the risk of serious physical, emotional, and professional consequences, including errors at work, damaged relationships, and even loss of licensure or employment. Recognizing a need for help and taking action is a sign of strength and a crucial step toward sustainable resilience and success, personally, professionally, and as an organization.

Organizations that continue to blame individuals for inadequate resilience in a culture that includes trauma exposure and chronic emotional strain will suffer from poor performance and teamwork, burnout, failure to retain and develop talent, absenteeism, presenteeism, and problematic team dynamics that fester over time.

Within my framework, I provide you with clear definitions, highlighting risk factors and symptoms, and offering evidence-based strategies. I am providing vital resources for both individuals and organizations striving to foster resilience and well-being in high-stress environments.

The need for trauma-informed workplaces and self-care is universal. In The ABELLA Model, you will discover it is more than a framework—it's a lifeline. This is one of the most common threads underlying what *looks like* burnout, over functioning, anxiety, addiction, underperformance, and sudden changes in behavior of formerly exemplary employees.

At home, the effects of trauma erode a person and their relationships insidiously over time, yet we almost never *talk* about what constitutes trauma and what kinds of jobs and roles increase exposure—it goes well beyond the cultural conversation across sectors and responsibility levels. Of course, helping professionals are highly susceptible, but so are leaders, lawyers, administrators, and those who have to process traumatic content, even vicariously.

I designed this book to feel like a conversation with me, your trusted mentor, packed with insights, real-world strategies, and moments of recognition that will make you pause, reflect, and take the next step forward.

Professionals who experience trauma, vicarious trauma, compassion fatigue, or burnout—and do not take steps to address it—may pay devastating consequences in their careers, relationships, and health and wellness.

But there is hope, and transformation is possible. If I could move from being shaped by trauma, self-medicating, and negativity (and believe me, I was deep in it for quite a while) to someone who now is in a much better place—someone who embraces growth, resilience, and a positive outlook—then you, too, can rewrite your story.

The journey may not be easy, but with the right tools and support, profound change is within reach.

In the next chapter, you'll discover how The ABELLA Model gives you a clear, step-by-step path to overcome these challenges—empowering you to reclaim your well-being, revitalize your leadership, and inspire meaningful change in yourself and your organization.

Let's walk this path together.

THE ABELLA MODEL™

It was about 4 am, and there was a knock on my door. I opened the door and saw him standing there, completely drenched in blood from head to toe. His eyes were bloodshot from crying, and he couldn't utter a word. I immediately started screaming, "Oh my God, no, no, no."

The night before, my police academy class celebrated our first anniversary of graduating from the LAPD academy at a restaurant in Pasadena. Afterwards, a few of us drove to my home in Hollywood to drink and party more. It was November 17, 1981.

Sometime after 2:00 a.m., one of the female officers, who was very drunk, wanted to drive home from Hollywood to the San Fernando Valley. All of us knew that she was too drunk to drive home. We tried to stop her. We took her keys away from her. We held her back and told her she was in no condition to drive. This went on for a while. As time went on, she seemed to finally give in, and we thought she would not drive, spend the night at my house, and drive home in the morning when she was sober.

However, at some point, she grabbed the keys from another officer's hand and ran out the door. She got into her car and drove away at a high rate of speed. A male officer jumped into his car and followed her. After driving about 20 miles, she tried to exit the freeway and flew off the embankment at a high rate of speed. The male officer, who had been following her the entire time, exited his vehicle and tried to rescue her, but she had been killed upon impact.

I had joined the Los Angeles Police Department (LAPD) as a brand-new academy recruit, only 21 years of age. It is a day I will never forget. We were the first class in which the height requirement was lowered from 5'6" to 5'0" to satisfy Francon Blake's consent decree as a result of a lawsuit against the City of Los Angeles for failing to recruit and hire a sufficient number of women and minorities. What I experienced going through the LAPD academy was one of the most grueling, exhausting, and demanding experiences of my life. I had never been in a quasi-military environment, and it was physically, mentally, emotionally, and intellectually demanding. Only about 40 of our initial 80 recruits made it through my academy class. Those who graduated had a very strong bond.

Dealing with the guilt, shock, grief, anxiety, and loss of a friend and colleague so early in my career left a huge mark. Every year on November 17th, I always think about my academy classmate and pray for her and her family. I know that she is in heaven with our Lord. This is just one of many traumatic events that I have had to live with throughout my life.

My life has had many ups and downs. I had a very abusive mother who constantly beat me. Back in the day, it was common for parents to whip, beat, slap, and punch their children as punishment, but the kind of beatings I received from my mom back then would constitute felony child abuse today.

To get away from my abusive mother, I got married at the age of 17. I went from the frying pan and jumped into the fire! My husband, who was seven years older than I, turned out to be a drug addict from "The Rock" in Tujunga. I was the victim of domestic violence.

I divorced him at the age of 21 and joined the LAPD. Again, frying pan to fire, this time much more psychological and social abuse. When I was on the LAPD, I did not know how to cope with all of the awful things I saw and experienced, so I did what all of the other patrol officers, my training officers, and supervisors did—and that was to drink. It was commonplace to drink alcohol to numb the pain.

I drank a lot when I was in the LAPD, because getting drunk was the only way I knew to "forget" all of the horrendous events and unspeakable horrors I witnessed.

Not only was I dealing with the atrocious realities I saw on the job with the public as a law enforcement officer, but there was severe and pervasive sexual harassment, sexual discrimination, racial discrimination, hostile work environment, and so many other types of unwelcome workplace conduct as part of the culture of the police force. Back in the 1980s, it was still a mostly white, male-dominated workforce.

During this time, neither the officers in the department nor the community members were accustomed to seeing female officers. Many of the male officers constantly "hit on us," always touching us, grabbing our butts, and brushing up against our breasts. Others treated us like slaves, making us shine their shoes, get their coffee, write all the reports, and do all of the usual tasks "females were made for." Even the public hit on us. There were numerous times, I would be driving on the street in my black and white police car, and guys would come up to me at a stop sign and say, "Hey, beautiful! Take me to jail. I want to be handcuffed to you!" I even had suspects I arrested ask for my phone number. *Are you kidding me?*

There were so many awful, horrific, and degrading experiences that I had to see and deal with. At that time, there were many situations I had simply blocked out so that I would never have to think about them again, because it caused panic attacks to recall them.

Now don't get me wrong, in my 20 years on the LAPD, I had a lot of wonderful memories working with certain officers, at certain divisions and/or assignments, and the community. My favorite division to work at was Wilshire Division. I loved being in law enforcement, loved helping others, and met so many wonderful people. This career has its ups and downs, good and bad. That's how it gets into you. It's plausible that some careers develop a sort of trauma bond to you.

While on the LAPD, I met my second husband, who was also a police officer. I was married again at the age of 28. Unfortunately, there were some of the same issues as in my first marriage and a few new ones. When he drank, it was like living with Dr. Jekyll and Mr. Hyde. I filed for divorce two years later. We tried to work things out. Our son was born, and we got back together, but the marriage didn't last, and I filed for divorce again. So by the age of 32, I had gone through three very costly divorces, which caused a lot of stress and anxiety. Fortunately, because of our son and the great relationship I have with his family, my second husband and I have remained friends, and we now have a good relationship. We spend all of the holidays together with our son, the step-kids, step-grandkids, and his family, whom I love very much. I could not have created this reality with my second husband if I had not addressed the issues in my life that came from trauma and created some real negative coping and survival patterns. After leaving the LAPD, I filed several lawsuits against the City of Los Angeles for various labor, employment, and civil rights allegations. Unfortunately, I was not well represented in one of those matters. I was devastated. I hired a malpractice attorney and filed a lawsuit against one of the attorneys who let me down, which I won, and that gave me the impetus to go to law school. I wanted to make sure that I would not get screwed over again, so I learned the law.

At the same time, I started my own business as a licensed private investigator. I started out conducting criminal defense cases, working on behalf of "alleged" murderers, rapists, and other hardcore criminals—this work made me sick to my stomach because I had put these types of people in prison for the past 20 years. (Sorry to all legal professionals who perform criminal defense work.) I transitioned to workers' compensation defense, which wasn't nearly as traumatic, but vicarious trauma from the content still crept into my psyche. I started to understand how pervasive this threat is to mental health in multiple professions.

If you fail to recognize the early warning signs of mental health issues, then the potential for significant physical, mental, and emotional decline increases. If your organization fails to cultivate a deeply trauma-informed culture and instead treats cumulative trauma as "just part of the job," then you risk compounding harm.

The ABELLA Model of Awareness, Blame, Evaluate, Learn, Leverage, and Action is different because many frameworks focus either on organizational policies or individual self-care, but rarely bridge both. My framework works when others fail because it acknowledges the "Why Now" factor, leverages existing support systems, validates without victimizing, and is scalable to organizations.

Amplify Awareness

At the outset, professionals must first recognize and confront avoidance. Avoidance often manifests as rationalizing unhealthy coping mechanisms or viewing burnout and compassion fatigue as inevitable job hazards. By refusing to acknowledge personal vulnerability or seek help, individuals remain stuck in ineffective patterns. By accepting and becoming aware of the problems, one must be able to "face it, in order to fix it."

Only by facing reality and accepting the need for change can professionals lay the groundwork for healthier, more sustainable work lives—and begin their journey toward resilience.

Organizations can support this step by fostering open communication and normalizing discussions about stress and trauma, creating a culture where acknowledging challenges is encouraged rather than stigmatized.

Beyond Blame

Secondly, my framework addresses the tendency to blame

external factors—such as colleagues, clients, or the system— and the shame for their personal distress, rather than examining one's own responses and needs.

This mindset often reinforces the "suck it up" mentality. This mentality tends to go with certain workplace cultures and values, brought in by the personality types and socialization patterns of people who are drawn to working in those sectors and roles.

Breaking free from blame and shame is essential because it allows individuals to take ownership of their well-being and recognize the real, personal consequences of trauma exposure. By shifting from blame and shame to accountability, professionals empower themselves to seek solutions and support, moving beyond resentment toward constructive action.

Organizations can help by promoting shared responsibility and facilitating structured opportunities for team feedback and reflection.

Examine and Evaluate

Surfacing the truth of how you are living today requires a thorough and honest self-assessment of your mental, emotional, and physical well-being. Here, professionals are encouraged to recognize warning signs of trauma-related stress and reflect on the effectiveness of their current coping strategies (or lack thereof). This critical evaluation helps individuals understand the risks of inaction—such as work errors, strained relationships, and declining health—and motivates them to pursue positive change. Without this honest appraisal, meaningful progress toward resilience and recovery is impossible. Organizations can implement regular well-being check-ins and provide access to confidential self-assessment tools to help staff monitor their health and stress levels.

Listen and Learn

Now that the individual has recognized the signs and symptoms and the "light is on," individuals actively seek knowledge about these issues and best practices for self-care and trauma-informed approaches. This step is about expanding awareness, identifying personal triggers, and discovering effective coping strategies through ongoing education and training. Learning equips professionals with the tools they need to manage stress and advocate for themselves and others. It is a vital step toward empowerment, enabling individuals to make informed decisions and build resilience. Organizations can foster continuous learning by offering workshops, training sessions, and resources on trauma-informed care and resilience-building.

Link and Leverage

Moving forward by linking the next step, focuses on leveraging available resources—such as peer support, supervision, professional help, and organizational tools—to strengthen resilience and well-being. Professionals are encouraged to build and maintain robust support networks with family, friends, and colleagues, and to implement self-care practices like proper sleep, nutrition, exercise, and mindfulness. Advocating for reasonable workloads and trauma-informed workplace policies is also key.

By leveraging these supports, individuals create a sustainable foundation for personal and professional growth, ensuring they are better equipped to handle ongoing challenges. Organizations can support this by providing access to employee assistance programs, peer support groups, and flexible policies that prioritize well-being.

Apply Action represents the culmination of The ABELLA Model, where professionals achieve resilience, balance, and a renewed sense of purpose by attaining a plan of action. By consistently applying trauma-informed strategies in both their personal and professional life, individuals become role models and resources for others in high-stress fields.

This final step fosters a positive, empathetic, and effective organizational culture, promoting fulfillment, well-being, and ongoing growth. Applying action means not only thriving personally but also contributing to the well-being of colleagues and the broader community, embodying the principles of trauma-informed leadership and advocacy. Organizations can reinforce this step by recognizing and rewarding resilience, facilitating mentorship programs, and modeling trauma-informed leadership at all levels.

The ABELLA Model is designed for individuals and leaders who have moved beyond denial and are genuinely ready to confront the realities of trauma, burnout, and emotional strain in their lives and workplaces. They are ready to find out what their work culture and engagement can feel like with people who are healing and fully living in the present.

This model is for those who not only recognize their own struggles but are also committed to transformation, willing to embrace support, challenge old patterns, and take meaningful action toward resilience and well-being for themselves and others in the places where they live and work.

The ABELLA Model is not for those who are still firmly entrenched in denial, unwilling to acknowledge the impact of trauma, burnout, or emotional strain in their lives or workplaces, who believe that greater coping is all that is required in order to perform consistently in a demanding role that carries a higher than average level of trauma exposure.

Remember, the workplace is not the only place a person likely finds exposure to trauma, but when they get it at work in addition to the world at large, it has a significant impact on an individual's mental and physical health, affecting their ability to function both at work and in their personal life.

If you are not yet ready to examine your own experiences, challenge long-held assumptions, or accept that change is possible—or if you believe that seeking help or support is a sign of weakness—this framework may feel overwhelming or unwelcome at this stage. I understand, and I urge you not to sit in overwhelm. Seek help, because it's out there.

However, if you already sense a growing awareness or curiosity, or if you are beginning to question the status quo, you may find that this model becomes a valuable resource when you are ready to take the next step toward growth and resilience.

In order to succeed, you will need to let go of the belief that you must always "suck it up", "that's part of the job," or that vulnerability is a sign of weakness. You need to at least consider challenging the assumption that self-medicating is a necessary coping mechanism. I urge you to move away from blaming others or the system for your struggles and instead recognize the importance of personal responsibility and self-care.

In other words, I'm asking you to abandon the idea that time alone will heal trauma. It doesn't.

During my years on the LAPD, I thought that as time went on, I would get accustomed to dealing with all these issues. I will "toughen up," have "thicker skin," "become strong," and to a certain point, you do. You learn how to project "command presence" when dealing with a suspect who is twice your size and could probably kill you with one punch. You learn how to walk, talk, and act confidently and take charge, especially as a supervisor. But there will always be certain situations in which unresolved memories can trigger intense reactions long after an event has occurred. This is where proactive interventions such as trauma-informed practices are of the utmost importance.

Breaking free from these outdated norms—such as neglecting self-care, overextending yourselves, or avoiding help due to stigma—will be crucial for lasting recovery and resilience. Adopting a growth mindset will empower you to see challenges as opportunities for learning and growth, rather than insurmountable obstacles. No more thinking "this is just the way it is." Things can change, and so can you. Thinking with self-compassion and self-awareness will help you recognize your own needs and take proactive steps toward healing.

You will also benefit from a proactive, action-oriented approach that values seeking support and setting healthy boundaries. Embracing a trauma-informed perspective—viewing trauma as a whole-person experience—and cultivating a collaborative mindset will further support your journey through The ABELLA Model toward resilience, well-being, and professional success.

Forward-thinking leaders who understand that their teams are vulnerable to these challenges and who are prepared to champion change, foster open dialogue, and create environments where growth and healing are possible, because they know that true strength comes from courage, self-awareness, and the willingness to seek and offer help, will also succeed.

Each step in The ABELLA Model builds on the one before it, ensuring that individuals and organizations move from denial and avoidance, through honest self-assessment and learning, toward leveraging support and ultimately thriving. Skipping steps risks leaving unresolved trauma, reinforcing harmful beliefs, or missing essential self-awareness and resources needed for true recovery and resilience. Completing each step in order allows for a strong foundation, steady progress, and lasting transformation, both personally and professionally, for the individual and the organization.

Each step of The ABELLA Model is essential. Once you have completed them in order, you're ready to embark on a journey that will challenge your deepest assumptions and open new doors to healing.

In the next chapter, we'll shine a light on the very first obstacle many professionals face: the powerful force of Amplifying Awareness. Together, we'll uncover why so many struggle to acknowledge their pain, explore the hidden costs of denial, and set the stage for real change.

If you've ever wondered what keeps you stuck or silent, get ready to find out, and prepare to take your first step toward lasting resilience.

To deepen your understanding and apply the insights from this chapter, I invite you to visit **www.LitaAbella.com** and use the interactive journal with seven guided questions—designed to help you reflect, plan, and take action on your journey toward resilience and well-being.

STEP ONE

Amplify Awareness

As I write this book, I can't help but wonder why things have not changed, especially when it comes to careers such as first responders. With the evolution of psychology and wellness, there still seems to be an ongoing and pervasive "suck it up" mentality among certain fields and acceptance of occupational hazards that are intrinsic to helping or public safety work.

Blindness seems to be acceptable in certain areas of the workforce until brave ones step forward and demand that their mental health be paid attention to.

I can see how cultural differences in certain fields make for a harder time accepting that things need to change. Law enforcement seems to be one of them. In April 1992, I vividly recall working the Los Angeles riots, which erupted when three LAPD police officers and one LAPD sergeant were acquitted for the "alleged" beating of Rodney King. At that time, I was married to a police officer but at a different division, and our son was only 18 months old. The entire LAPD was mobilized, which meant that all days off were canceled. We had to work 12-hour shifts every day. There was a curfew in effect in the city of Los Angeles.

My then-husband and I worked opposite shifts, but our son's nanny quit when I asked her to work some extra hours and days due to our emergency mandatory schedules. I had no space to make alternate arrangements, so I ended up taking my son to work with me and giving him to the desk officers to watch while I gave roll call to the officers.

For women, it's a double whammy. If you scoff at that, you may be part of the problem.

For weeks, we barely hung on, sleeping only if our son slept, passing him back and forth like a baton. No one's needs were met. It was awful driving through the city of LA with all the mayhem, rioting, burning buildings, shootings, looting, fights, and chaos everywhere, especially with my son in the car.

What is so ironic, as I write this book, is that we are experiencing a very similar situation. I still live in LA County, and because of the political climate, there are numerous protests for various reasons in LA County as well as surrounding counties. Unfortunately, the protests have turned into riots, the national guard and the marines have been summoned to Southern California, and LA County has been under a curfew in sections of downtown LA for the past several days. I can well imagine what law enforcement and the first responders are dealing with mentally, physically, and emotionally. I lived it, thirty-three years ago.

These traumatic events are just a few months after the horrendous, devastating, and deadly fires in Pacific Palisades and Altadena in Los Angeles County, and then the mudslides a month after that. Law enforcement and the first responders have been on a continuous roller coaster of traumatic events with no downtime to process these incidents, and many of them were victims of the fires, floods, and mudslides as well.

What has changed with the organizations?

Law enforcement and first responders? Legal and criminal justice professionals?

Not much.

Law enforcement officers, firefighters, and other first responders have to put their lives on hold to serve the public. Deputy district attorneys, public defenders, victim advocates, and other criminal justice and legal professionals have their case loads doubled or tripled and are expected to deal with it all and, again, "suck it up."

The organizations, government agencies, and other public service entities have to respond to the public's needs, but there doesn't appear to be anything in place to help the public servants who are there for the community members. At times such as these, organizations failed to acknowledge the reality and the set of problems that arise when this happens.

When something terrible happens, such as suicides among law enforcement officers, or a first responder falling asleep while driving because of severe sleep deprivation, or a spouse who goes home and beats his wife and/or children because he "snapped" due to the stress and trauma he has been dealing with, fingers point in many different directions deflecting the blame and shame. No one will take responsibility, especially the organizations/government agencies, because they answer to their constituents (the voting public). Thus, it's best not to acknowledge that there is a problem until it is too late.

In the entire 20 years that I was on the LAPD, I was not aware of the mental health issues I was dealing with. I avoided (really ignored) these issues by keeping myself extremely busy. My life was a constant "Go, Go, Go," such that 20 years went by in a flash. I was so engrossed with my "faster, bigger, and more" career on the LAPD that for a long while, I couldn't remember anything about my son's childhood. I only spent the first six months of his life with him, which I enjoyed tremendously. I loved being a mom, and my son was (and still is) my entire world.

I loved spending every minute of every day with him during his first six months of life, but once I returned to work from maternity leave, it seemed that the next time I recall engaging with my son was in 2000, when I left the LAPD, and by then, my son was 10 years old!

I know that in reality, that is not true. I know I spent quality time with him, but for some reason, I don't have any vivid memories of him when he was young. All I remember was dropping my son off with my mom, a babysitter, or pre-school, and then school. By then, we didn't have a nanny living with us, which we had off and on throughout his young life.

Where did all the time go?

Why did I let my life slip away from me?

There are so many situations that I have blocked out of my mind because they were so difficult to endure. As a result, I buried the good along with any awareness that I wasn't functioning at my best, being present to my life on an everyday level. I am shocked at what a blur it looks like in the rearview mirror. I was on autopilot and almost the last to know it, because I was psychologically and emotionally in survival mode for so long.

Most professionals around me who were dealing with these issues would also ignore the problem, attempt to hide it from family, friends, and colleagues, and remind themselves to "suck it up" and not complain because it is part of the job —and that is what I did for years. These fields are also isolating, so your circle of relationships revolves around people with the same set of problems and problematic coping skills.

"Awareness is the greatest agent for change."—Eckhart Tolle.

It is hard to come forward and admit there is a problem and that you need help, especially in the "helping others" industries, wherein the public comes to us for help. It is part of the culture to be in denial about it or to blame the job or the circumstances, and not believe there is a solution. If you are the helper, who would you think of *to help you?*

When I was deep into avoidance of the issue, my coping skills amounted to alcohol and overwork, and there was a long period of time before anything interrupted that. It was all normalized by the environment and culture. Yet it was far from healthy or sustainable.

At the heart of every journey toward healing and resilience is the willingness to face what's real, especially when reality is painful, uncomfortable, or frightening. For professionals in high-stress, trauma-exposed fields, surfacing some awareness of what you are blocking, avoiding, soothing, or afraid to re-experience is often the first and most formidable barrier to progress. It is a natural human instinct: When confronted with overwhelming stress, trauma, or emotional strain, our minds and bodies urge us to turn away, to deny, or to minimize what we're experiencing. While avoidance may offer temporary relief, it ultimately traps us in cycles of suffering, isolation, and stagnation.

Avoidance takes many forms. For some, it's denying the impact of traumatic events or daily stressors, pretending everything is "fine" even as exhaustion and emotional pain accumulate. For others, it's rationalizing unhealthy coping mechanisms— self-medicating with alcohol and/or drugs, being a workaholic, or withdrawal—as "normal" or even "deserved" indulgences or excuses given the demands of the job. Still others believe that burnout, compassion fatigue, and vicarious trauma are simply the price of admission for their chosen careers, and that accepting awareness and being vulnerable or reaching out for support is often seen as admitting defeat. This mindset is reinforced by workplace cultures that equate strength with silence and resilience with stoicism.

The consequences of unchecked avoidance are profound. Research shows that avoiding trauma memories or reminders impedes the natural recovery process, preventing individuals from habituating to distressing experiences and allowing heightened arousal to persist. Over time, avoidance can reinforce PTSD symptoms by signaling to the brain that trauma memories are dangerous and must be avoided at all costs.

In the context of burnout and compassion fatigue, avoidance

leads to emotional, physical, and mental exhaustion, as individuals suppress their needs and push through pain until they reach a "breaking point." This not only harms the individual but also erodes team morale, productivity, and the overall health of organizations.

Not accepting awareness is not just a personal challenge— it's a systemic one. When *organizations* fail to foster open communication about stress and trauma—or when they stigmatize vulnerability—they inadvertently reinforce avoidance behaviors. Employees learn that it's safer to keep quiet, to "suck it up," and to avoid drawing attention to their struggles. This creates a culture where suffering is hidden, support is underutilized, and preventable crises escalate. The result is a workforce that is less resilient, less engaged, and more prone to turnover, absenteeism, and errors.

Everyone has different "breaking points." For some, it could mean I need to step back, take a look at my life, and really think about what this type of work is doing to me and my family. For others, it is leaving a job that you once loved for another career that provides a better work-life balance. For others, it could be finding maladaptive behaviors such as self-medicating with alcohol and/or drugs. For others, it could be ending your life.

According to an article in the Daily Journal, "Ferguson's Murder Conviction Exposes Gaps in California's Judicial Oversight", dated April 28, 2025, by Douglas Saunders Sr., stated, "Ferguson, a longtime (Orange County, CA) deputy district attorney and a (Orange County, CA) Superior Court judge for 10 years, drank during work hours—with colleagues and members of the bar— and carried a weapon on the bench, according to trial testimony." No one wanted to acknowledge what was going on and turned a blind eye, and avoided confronting and/or reporting this judge. Ferguson, age 74, was convicted of second-degree murder for the Aug. 3, 2023, shooting death of his wife during an alcohol-fueled domestic dispute. The shooting took place in their home in front of their 22-year-old son. Ferguson faces 40 years to life in prison. *As of this writing, Ferguson is still awaiting sentencing.*

According to the article in The Current Report, "Another Suicide at LASD (Los Angeles Sheriff's Department): The Body Count Rises to 13 Under Sheriff Luna", dated May 18, 2025, written by Cece Woods, there have been 13 suicides in 17 months since Robert Luna became the Sheriff. Moreover, during a 24-hour period in November 2023, four lives were lost. According to a letter released in response to the November suicides, it stated, "We work multiple overtime shifts a week, often only getting a couple of hours of sleep between continuous double shifts... We are frequently denied time off ... Our leadership sides with criminals while condemning us."

According to this article, and from the numerous LAPD officers that I personally knew and who died by suicide, it would lead one to believe that these law enforcement officers reached their "breaking point" and made the decision to end their lives. No one will ever know what specifically led them to make that ultimate decision, but being in a constant state of overwhelm, burnout, anxiety, depression, and other mental health issues was most likely a contributing factor.

Having knowledge is power. Understanding and being able to identify and acknowledge that something is wrong, and not ignoring the situation, is a start. Being able to talk about these issues is a step in the right direction.

You can't even begin to talk about it until you are willing to look at it. The deeper excavation is where so many people hold back. Where organizations fail to go beyond the surface to acknowledge what their employees and leadership are carrying within, from the subject matter and sensory inputs they have been exposed to in the role.

If you fail to recognize the early warning signs of mental health issues, then the potential for significant physical, mental, and emotional decline increases.

If your organization fails to cultivate a deeply trauma-informed culture and instead treats cumulative trauma as "just part of the job," then you risk compounding harm.

When individuals are working too much without proper time off to recharge and process some of the traumatic events they have dealing with on a daily basis, dealing with unreasonable caseloads, and working with little to no resources such as insufficient staff, mistakes will be make, customer service will be poor, there will be high turnover, low morale, more staff calling in sick, people suffering from illnesses or injuries which could result in long term leave of absence, and the ultimate is death or suicides.

If you ignore the warning signs, then you fail to acknowledge that a challenge is present.

If you ignore the signs of trauma and stress in your workforce, then you fail to raise awareness of the real challenges your team faces.

Individuals and organizations must stop avoiding and start

working through the problem because history is going to repeat itself generation after generation.

Blame is the second step because, after achieving awareness that a problem exists, it is common for individuals—and even organizations—to react by attributing the issue to others, the system, or external factors rather than examining their own role or needs. This step of blaming serves as a natural defense mechanism, but also highlights an important moment for growth: by recognizing and moving past blame, you begin to shift toward personal and collective accountability, which is essential for meaningful change.

Avoiding awareness traps individuals in denial, normalizes harmful coping mechanisms (e.g., substance use), and fosters shame. Without acknowledging the problem, unresolved trauma intensifies, leading to emotional detachment, cynicism, or explosive anger. Unaddressed issues can manifest as job errors, licensure loss, relationship breakdowns, or health crises.

If you skip the Amplify Awareness step, then you cannot break the (cycle of) Blame, Evaluate risks honestly, or Leverage solutions, resulting in systemic failure for individuals and organizations.

Why, then, is amplifying awareness the critical first step? Only by facing reality—by acknowledging the impact of stress, trauma, and emotional strain—can professionals begin to heal and grow.

Awareness is an act of courage and self-efficacy. It means admitting that you are human, that you are affected by your experiences, and that you deserve support and care. It means challenging the myth that vulnerability is weakness and embracing the truth that it is the foundation of true strength and resilience.

Amplifying awareness opens the door to every other step in The ABELLA Model. It allows individuals to move beyond denial and blame, to honestly evaluate their well-being, and to seek the knowledge and resources they need to thrive.

For organizations, raising awareness means creating environments where open dialogue about mental health is encouraged, where support is accessible and destigmatized, and where leaders model vulnerability and self-care. This shift not only benefits individuals but also strengthens the entire team, fostering a culture of trust, empathy, and shared growth.

Awareness is the gateway to transformation. It is the moment when professionals and leaders decide to stop running from pain and start facing it—not alone, but with the support and resources that make healing possible. By amplifying awareness, you lay the groundwork for a healthier, more sustainable work life, and you take the first essential step on the path to resilience, purpose, and lasting well-being.

I hope you now understand why you cannot continue to actively ignore or minimize your trauma symptoms. You must acknowledge and accept the problem.

Acceptance occurs here as you transition from externalizing responsibility ("My job causes this...") to internal acknowledgement ("This is my reality ..."). The next section dismantles blame-shifting—whether directed at institutions, colleagues, or yourself—by demonstrating how blame perpetuates stagnation. You will accept your situation when you stop attributing suffering solely to external factors.

To deepen your understanding and apply the insights from this chapter, I invite you to visit **www.LitaAbella.com** and use the interactive journal with seven guided questions—designed to help you reflect, plan, and take action on your journey toward resilience and well-being.

STEP TWO

Beyond Blame

I just returned home from a week-long empowerment business conference with so many engaging speakers. I vividly recall one of the speakers, a family doctor from San Diego, CA. She discussed her story of wanting to become a doctor and the profound impact of physicians on her own family's life growing up. She had no idea about the culture of medicine and how it would impact her and her family.

She explained how her internship was the typical 80-hour work week. She was working non-stop, 24/7, and developed focal neurologic symptoms, which progressed to status epilepticus—a prolonged seizure or a series of seizures without regaining consciousness between them—due to sleep deprivation. She ended up intubated, comatose, and nonresponsive for a week.

When she finally woke up, her future was unclear. Her doctors didn't think she could finish residency due to likely anoxic brain injury, which occurs when the brain receives no oxygen at all. She ended up becoming a full clinical professor, director of multiple programs, and an awarded medical educator.

She had it all, the family, the career, and was on top of the world—but thanks to the pervasive messages she'd received early in her career about what "normal" for a doctor would look like, she didn't realize she was a "workaholic." She had a bike accident in 2017, and that was her "breaking point." In her recovery from the accident, she finally stopped avoiding her mental health issues and acknowledged there was a problem. She finally recognized that things in her life had to change.

"When you blame others, you give up your power to change."
— Dr. Robert Anthon.

Blame occurs when individuals attribute their struggles to others, the system, or external circumstances, rather than addressing their own reactions and needs. In an individual, this can look like "tough" behavior, chronic conflict, or apparent resilience, but it's a false resilience based on bypassing or false "acceptance" of the *futility* of change. In a group, this often manifests as a "suck it up" mentality, where strength is equated with silence and resilience is misunderstood.

It was common in the medical field for doctors to work 80-hour workweeks caring for their patients. But it wasn't until this doctor experienced two near-death experiences of her own that she finally recognized that she—and her lifestyle norms—contributed directly to her health issues, even including being accident-prone from fatigue and mental fog.

Overcoming blame means accepting that trauma exposure has real personal consequences and that seeking support is a sign of true strength.

In the legal profession, I see, read about, and talk with many attorneys who work in "Big Law." It is very prestigious, and they get paid very well, but most attorneys have no work-life balance. They eat, drink, and live for their career, especially when working as a trial attorney. Many wish their job didn't consume the majority of their time each day, and dream of a life where they can come home and not continue to work until the early morning hours. They know that in order to have a successful career, they have to put everything else aside and make their career their number one priority. Everything else and everyone else, including their family, has to take a back seat.

To cope with this stressful life, they start self-medicating, and alcohol is usually the most common way to self-medicate. When their life starts to crumble, things start to fall between the cracks, they are irritable due to sleep deprivation, their spouse and children complain that they are never home and/or never pay any attention to them, the individual starts to point fingers at everyone and everything else but themselves. They feel that on top of this "extreme job," they should not have normal demands placed upon them, and they get resentful, impatient, and detached.

I have been in very similar situations in my 45-year career, and I empathize with those of you in the same or similar scenarios. But after all the finger-pointing and the blame and shame, one thing you must remember is that you have control of your own life.

If you are in a toxic situation that is causing harm to your physical, emotional, and/or mental health, you retain the power to walk away.

So often, we receive social messages that it's never okay to quit or to give up, or that we have a duty to stand up for injustice. (Well, maybe that last one was me, and it sure took me a long time to put that burden down when it became too big to carry.) Maybe you need to take a break, take a step back, and reassess, or maybe it is time to move on to a better and brighter life in a different area of practice, or maybe a different industry.

Blame naturally follows avoidance in the healing and resilience process. When individuals begin to move away from denial and start acknowledging their struggles, the next instinct is often to search for a cause or a culprit—either internal or external—to explain their pain and distress. This is a normal psychological response: after confronting the discomfort that comes with facing reality, people may look for something or someone to hold responsible for their suffering. Blame, whether directed at oneself ("I should have done more") or others ("They didn't support me"), can feel like a way to regain a sense of control in the chaos of trauma and stress.

Imagine, after a difficult loss in court, a young trial attorney might initially avoid acknowledging the emotional toll of the outcome. As the weight of the loss settles in, they begin to blame others or the system: "If the judge had ruled differently," or "If my client had been more cooperative, we would have won." They may even turn blame inward, thinking, "I should have prepared better," or "I'm not cut out for this."

In this stage, the attorney is caught in a cycle of frustration and self-doubt, focusing on what went wrong and who is at fault, rather than reflecting on what they can learn or how they can grow from the experience. This is the Blame step in action for a new trial attorney—a necessary, but transitional, phase before self-evaluation and resilience can truly begin.

You may have to walk through the fire to get to the other side. There are many people who have encountered similar challenges as the ones described above and have lived to tell their stories, and many have wonderful, thriving, and resilient lives. Overcoming challenges and moving beyond blame helps us to learn, grow, and become stronger.

If you fail to recognize the early warning signs of mental health issues, then the potential for significant physical, mental, and emotional decline increases; therefore, knowing the strategies for dealing with these issues is crucial for your effective coping and recovery.

Too many helping professionals are constantly in survival mode and just trying to get through the next day, suppressing all the most difficult realities and emotional experiences they have along the way.

If your organization fails to cultivate a deeply trauma-informed culture and instead treats cumulative trauma as "just part of the job," then you risk compounding harm, diminishing the effectiveness and well-being of your professionals, increasing liability and staff turnover, and ultimately undermining your mission to serve with true empathy and effectiveness.

Insanity, by definition, is doing the same things all over again and expecting a different result. Too many organizations are insane when it comes to trauma: expecting individuals to handle it on their own, or not have to handle it at all.

If you move Beyond Blame, then you unlock the ability to

collaborate, learn, and move forward—both individually and as an organization.

However, blame is a double-edged sword. While it may offer temporary relief by providing a target for frustration or anger, it ultimately keeps individuals stuck in cycles of resentment, self-criticism, or hopelessness.

This is why The ABELLA Model places the Blame step before Evaluate: individuals must first recognize and move through their blaming tendencies before they can honestly and objectively assess their situation and begin to take meaningful action toward change. Organizations have to look for a blame-oriented culture and understand how that is counterproductive and prevents people from getting the support and care they deserve.

Without addressing blame, progress is limited—people remain trapped in a victim mindset, unable to reclaim agency over their own healing and growth.

Without addressing blame, individuals remain locked in unproductive patterns—such as resentment toward colleagues, systems, or themselves—preventing progress to honest self-evaluation and problem-solving. Blame fuels workplace conflict, eroding trust and collaboration. Teams become fractured, communication falters, and productivity declines as energy shifts from solutions to finger-pointing.

Organizations interpret this as a cultural problem and blame individuals for bringing in "personal drama," when it may actually have deep roots in the role they perform and the culture of the workplace itself.

Trauma survivors often will internalize blame on their own, leading to toxic self-criticism and feelings of unworthiness. This amplifies symptoms of PTSD, anxiety, and depression. The "suck it up" mentality—common in high-stress professions— accelerates burnout when someone's nervous system is too overwhelmed to cope and they are served what amounts to an invalidating and isolating sentiment. They tend to freeze and burn through their internal resources, struggling to properly place both the events that occurred and the shame and isolation they feel because it had an impact at all.

Suppressing emotions drains mental energy, leaving individuals feeling hollow and disconnected. Neurobiological research shows that unprocessed blame keeps the brain in survival mode.

Blame acts as a bridge between *avoidance* (denial) and *evaluation* (self-assessment). Without confronting blame, agency is lost: Individuals stay in a victim mindset, powerless to change their circumstances.

Moreover, growth stalls: Honest self-reflection becomes impossible, blocking the path to learning and leveraging resources.

The antidote to blame is to wholly accept the facts, circumstances, feelings, reactions, and situations you find yourself in, without judgment. You therefore start at your *honest* starting point. Not should, would, could, *if only*, but where you are today. If you feel ashamed that you didn't do better, it's likely that you couldn't do better until now. When you make peace with that reality, you stop the loop of self-flagellation that drives you back into the behaviors, thoughts, and patterns you no longer want.

In an organization, a blame culture must be pulled from the root wherever it takes form. Honoring the individuals who developed trauma-response type behavior from the exposures on the job is a way to uphold employee and leader well-being as a core value. We accept that this is to some degree inevitable, and we accept that it is a core function of the organization to address it.

In high-stress careers, bypassing blame isn't just a personal setback—it reinforces cultures of silence, where suffering goes unaddressed and resilience remains out of reach. This shows up in individual *and* organizational performance metrics and well-being. What if you could move beyond blame and reclaim your power to shape your own story? Imagine what becomes possible when you shift from pointing fingers to honestly exploring your own experiences and needs.

For example, imagine an attorney moving from "Big Law" to become a solo or small firm practitioner in an area of practice that she enjoys. Or a medical professional, leaving the 12 to 18-hour shifts in the emergency room and working every other weekend at the largest and busiest hospital in the County, to a solo practice in a small town where he knows his patients by their first and last name and is home by 6:00 p.m.

After I left the LAPD, I started my own firm as a licensed private investigator. It was great being an entrepreneur, working from home, creating my own hours, only answering to myself, and being able to go out and network and meet new people. I love being my own boss, not having to deal with anyone micro-managing me, and being accountable for all my successes as well as my failures, but being an entrepreneur, there is no one to point fingers at but yourself.

As you prepare to take this next step, ask yourself: What am I truly feeling right now—and what might I discover if I give myself permission to look inward? In the next chapter, you'll learn how honest self-evaluation–and acceptance *without* judgment–opens new pathways to resilience, well-being, and meaningful change.

To deepen your understanding and apply the insights from this chapter, I invite you to visit www.LitaAbella.com and use the interactive journal with seven guided questions—designed to help you reflect, plan, and take action on your journey toward resilience and well-being.

STEPS THREE & FOUR

Examine and Evaluate; Listen and Learn

When I worked at the State Bar of California, Office of Chief Trial Counsel, I investigated hundreds of attorneys who faced disciplinary action. Common threads among the majority of the attorneys I investigated were mostly solo or small firm practitioners who wore too many hats.

In other words, not only are they the attorney, but they are also the bookkeeper and accountant, HR manager, social media manager, marketing person, paralegal, and investigator. They were overwhelmed and suffering from burnout, trying to do everything in their firm. Needless to say, details get overlooked, critical items are neglected, and important tasks are missed, resulting in errors and quality can suffer. Some errors may be minor, but many resulted in serious misconduct.

Many of the attorneys that I talked to were also self-medicating with alcohol and/or drugs (including illegal and legal drugs), or some other addictive behavior such as food, gambling, pornography, or other dysfunctional means to cope with the mental health issues they may or may not have consciously known they were suffering from. The three most common mental health concerns among attorneys are depression, anxiety, and stress. This is true not only in the legal industry but in many other industries, such as healthcare.

The personal, ethical, and moral responsibility of professionals in high-stress jobs requires them to examine and evaluate when their job is affecting their physical, mental, or emotional health by knowing the signs and symptoms of the mental health issues they may develop in the course of their professional lives.

They would demonstrate accountability by doing something visible to resolve the issue such as (1) requesting a reduced caseload, taking time off, going to a medical and/or mental health professional, (2) ensuring that they are taking care of themselves by getting sufficient sleep, eating healthy meals, exercising, and practicing mindfulness, mediation, and/or gratitude, and (3) talking about these issues with family, friends, or colleagues.

In order for professionals in high-stress careers to be able to take care of their clients, their families, and themselves, they need to make sure they are healthy physically, mentally, and emotionally.

If they do not, this can lead to some devastating consequences and losses:

- Errors and other issues at work which could result in disciplinary action that could lead to a negative performance evaluation, suspension, termination, and/or loss of their professional license (such as disbarment for an attorney, medical license for a medical professional, loss of their peace officer status for law enforcement, etc.)

- Loss of reputation, loss of clients, and loss of income.

- Loss of the family unit, separation/divorce, loss of custody of their children, and an increase in financial obligations such as child or spousal support.

- Loss of their mental, physical, or emotional health would increase their financial obligations by paying high medical bills, etc.

- Serious bodily injury or death by getting into an accident because they were impaired/inattentive due to fatigue or being under the influence of alcohol and/or drugs.

- Suicide, due to job-related stress, burnout, mental health conditions, social isolation, work-life imbalance, access to lethal means, exposure to traumatic events, financial instability, job insecurity, and stigma around mental health.

- Homicide due to violent situations because of the profession (i.e., law enforcement), aggressive clients/patients/co-workers seeking revenge, or who may have been terminated or whose services have been terminated, resulting in the professional being killed and/or a mass shooting (military base, government offices, malls, schools, etc.).

However, the very first (and often missing) observation is that they have a problem they must solve—and that only they can do it. *No one* is coming to help the helper, and the culture of bypassing and "sucking up" invalidates the need for help. This step is all about reframing whose life this is, and who needs to step up and step in to make and actualize a change.

In an organization, this step is about understanding the trauma-driven roots of cultural dysfunction and performance problems and deciding to do something about it. For real this time, not just put it on the objectives for the year that never get funded or become part of the top ten must-dos. Putting it up near the top as a core responsibility makes it more likely that it becomes part of the operating system of the organization.

There was a time in my career when I avoided taking full responsibility for setbacks, sometimes blaming external circumstances or other people for the challenges I faced. Sometimes, I correctly blamed the culture of an organization for repeated events that caused me personal harm, but failed to take responsibility for removing *myself* from that situation the first time it became clear I could not make the organization change on my own.

This lack of accountability—not only the organization's, but my own for getting stuck in the "fight back" loop instead of the fully-processed acceptance pattern—slowly eroded my confidence and momentum, as I found myself stuck in the same responses, unable to move forward or learn from my experiences. The result was a sense of stagnation and diminished clarity about my goals, mirroring what research shows: Without accountability, progress stalls, and both personal and professional growth become elusive.

It just doesn't have to stay that way. When we become aware of ourselves, what we are avoiding and blaming for our pain, and that we have more options than we have been conditioned to see, we reclaim our own power and make it more accessible to ourselves for proper handling of the everyday little things as well as the big things that have caused us trauma along the way.

I've been where you are—trapped in cycles of blame and self-doubt, feeling stuck and uncertain about how to move forward. Know that this struggle is real, but it doesn't have to define your path or your potential for change. You are about to discover just how much power you really hold in the situation—and it's that personal power that you've lost sight of, and felt deprived of, for too long.

In this chapter, I discuss Step 3, Examine and Evaluate, and Step 4, Listen and Learn. They are inextricably linked as the phase of this model where the individual begins to take full responsibility for their own healing, recovery, and growth. Though they are separately named, the two are as both sides of a coin.

Step 3: Examine and Evaluate

"Without proper self-evaluation, failure is inevitable."—John Wooden.

This step is the cornerstone of accountability in The ABELLA Model. Until you have conducted an honest self-assessment of your mental, emotional, and physical well-being, you do not truly know your current reality. This self-assessment gives shape to things like identifying warning signs, ineffective coping strategies, and the tangible risks—or possibly emergent results—of your inaction to date (e.g., declining performance or health). This introspection demands ownership of one's state, transforming vague discomfort into actionable insights. Without this step, growth remains theoretical; accountability begins when we stop blaming external forces, circumstances, and events and instead ask, "What role do I play in my challenges, and what can I control?"

Step 4: Listen and Learn

"If you are not willing to learn, no one can help you. If you are determined to learn, no one can stop you."—Zig Ziglar.

Building on self-evaluation, this step embodies proactive accountability through humility and curiosity. Here, we seek knowledge and education that we may have never known existed, or applied to *ourselves*, about trauma, resilience, and evidence-based strategies. We broaden our horizons to allow room for change by listening to experts, peers, and research. Learning prepares us to recognize our own agency, equipping us with tools to address gaps identified in Step 3. For example, a social worker recognizing burnout (Step 3) might learn mindfulness techniques or boundary-setting (Step 4), shifting from "I'm terminally overwhelmed," to "Here's how I'll adapt and process each day so I can manage."

Examine and Evaluate must precede Listen and Learn because self-assessment creates the "why" for learning. That elucidates the gap. Without recognizing personal vulnerabilities or gaps (Step 3), learning lacks urgency and relevance.

When we can step off the "faster, bigger, more" hamster wheel of futility, which is one amusing way of describing how we behave when we do not believe we have the power to change anything about the job or the workplace that is exposing us to trauma, we see possibilities that we simply could not before.

For example, the Los Angeles City Fire Department (LAFD)

firefighter who has been working the Green shift, (LAFD firefighters work a "California shift," which is a 24-hour on, 24-hour off, 24-hour on, 24-hour off, 24-hour on, and then four days off) but now has a wife who is pregnant and bedridden because of certain medical issues: The firefighter realizes he needs to be home more with his wife to help manage the household. He seeks and gets an administrative job within the fire department that has a Monday-Friday, 8 am to 5 pm schedule so that he can be home more to support his wife and family and have a more manageable work-life balance. He knows he will be giving up all of the overtime pay, which could amount to a substantial amount of income, but can you put a price on you and your family's well-being?

Or the emergency room nurse who evaluates her symptoms from exhaustion, overwhelm, and burnout from working 12-hour shifts for the past several years (Step 3) and learns stress-management techniques such as exercise, proper nutrition, sufficient sleep, and practicing meditation (Step 4). After doing the work, she doesn't just "cope" anymore—she transforms her approach to work, modeling resilience for her colleagues. The change could be transferring to a medical facility that is closer to home, cutting her commute time from three hours each shift to one hour. The two hours she now saves are where she can incorporate an extra hour of sleep, 30 minutes for exercise, and 30 minutes for making healthy, nutritious meals to take to work.

It's true that most people do not change until they have to. This step is about surfacing and recognizing that there is a need to change, and noticing the urgency that we have created by attempting to ignore or bypass it for so long.

Organizations using this sequence foster cultures where employees drive their growth, reducing stigma around help-seeking and promoting sustainable well-being.

Transformation requires this sequence:

- Step 3 exposes the *need* for change (accountability for the present).

- Step 4 provides the *means* for change (accountability for the future).

- Together, they form a feedback loop: Evaluation reveals *what* to learn; Learning, in turn, refines future evaluations.

By grounding learning in self-evaluation, The ABELLA Model ensures accountability isn't punitive but empowering—turning insight into action, and action into lasting change.

If you avoid honestly examining your mental, emotional, and physical well-being, then you risk repeating unhelpful patterns and missing opportunities for meaningful change.

If you fail to listen to new perspectives, actively learn from experts, and acknowledge the truth about your experiences, you will continue to limit your ability to grow, adapt, and build true resilience.

Examine and Evaluate is the moment of honest self-assessment: It's about taking ownership of your current state, identifying gaps, and acknowledging the real risks of inaction. This step prevents denial or complacency, ensuring that individuals and organizations do not overlook the impacts of trauma and stress. Accountability here means facing the truth about what is—and isn't—working, which is the foundation for meaningful change.

When we stop looking elsewhere for something to change, we begin to reclaim our power to change the way we, and our workplaces, handle the reality of trauma and its effects on the people and workplaces we care about.

Listen and Learn builds on this by actively seeking out knowledge, strategies, and support to address those gaps. This step is about humility and openness—recognizing that growth comes from learning and applying new insights. Accountability in this context means committing to continuous improvement, which is essential for resilience and long-term success.

Together, these steps ensure that both individuals and organizations do not just passively acknowledge trauma and stress but take responsibility for addressing them. This accountability is what protects careers, reputations, and well-being, and it is what enables organizations to fulfill their missions with empathy and effectiveness. Without these steps, the risks of derailment, liability, and burnout remain unchecked; with them, transformation and sustainable success become possible and open the door for the next steps.

Accountability through honest evaluation and active learning lays the essential groundwork—identifying your needs and gathering the right tools—so you're ready to connect with resources and take effective action in the next steps.

When you truly own your growth in these ways, linking to support and achieving sustained change becomes not just possible, but powerful and purposeful. That's what the next step is about, the sustainable and (often accelerated) action to transform your wellbeing. This only happens once you have done all this preparation and worked through some essential practices to address the trauma. Why did it take you so long? Because you didn't know what you didn't know. After this, you have been taught the basic tools for overcoming traumatic patterns and actualizing personal change.

To deepen your understanding and apply the insights from this chapter, I invite you to visit **www.LitaAbella.com** and use the interactive journal with seven guided questions, designed to help you reflect, plan, and take action on your journey toward resilience and well-being.

STEPS FIVE & SIX

Link and Leverage; Apply Action

When the money ran out, I had two choices: either kill myself and get it all over with, or quit the LAPD and walk away with nothing. No pension, no retirement, no badge, no gun, no honor, nothing, nada. I was at my "breaking point" by then, and could not see anything good coming from fighting any longer.

I was dealing with so many issues. I loved my career in the LAPD, the community I served, and the excitement (and sometimes fun) of being in law enforcement, but I hated the BS and politics of the department.

I had always worked hard in every role I was assigned. I studied diligently, passed all the promotional exams, and worked my way up the ranks within the LAPD. Becoming one of the first female training officers who was allowed to train another female officer in Wilshire Division. This was unheard of back in the early 1980s! Back then, the "brass" (a.k.a. leadership) didn't think two females were competent enough to work together and that we would probably get ourselves killed in the field on patrol.

In another coveted assignment, my partner and I were one of the first undercover Vice teams that allowed two females to work together as partners in Southwest Division (South-Central LA).

I was the first female Sr. Lead Officer in patrol and one of the first female minority lieutenants in patrol. I worked on many different assignments and was promoted up the ranks of the LAPD relatively fast. Of course, the males (mostly male white officers and supervisors) alleged that the only reason I was promoted was because I was a minority female, "affirmative action," and all of the lawsuits filed against the department.

The higher I was promoted, the tougher things got.

I was more afraid of the knives stabbing me in the back by colleagues than I was of getting killed by a suspect on the streets.

As I stated earlier, I had filed several lawsuits against the LAPD for various labor, employment, and civil rights allegations. I was determined to hold people—and the department—accountable for egregious violations of equal employment and basic decency.

Of course, being willing to do the hard things comes at a price.

I worked in Northeast Division, a division that was known at that time for being anti-women and anti-Black, as a sergeant (June 1988-June 1989) and as a lieutenant (Sept. 1996 to Sept. 1997). I was told by my commanding officer that I was transferred to Northeast Division specifically because of the problems they were having. He hoped that my being one of the first female, minority sergeants (and subsequently one of the first female, minority lieutenants) would help reduce the disparate treatment females and minorities encounter there.

He had high hopes, and I admired him for that.

Whenever I was out in the field, I would be by myself because I was a supervisor. Working at night, it's easy to find suspects in the act of committing crimes. I would literally run into them. There were many times while I was working the graveyard shift that I would have to put out an "Officer Needs Back-Up, Assistance, or Help Call," and no one from Northeast Division would respond.

It was bewildering. Confusing. And dangerous.

I was even told by one of the "Old Timers" (who was also a sergeant), *"We don't like Blacks and we don't like women, you are on your own."*

I would pray that I wouldn't get killed. It would take several minutes, which seemed like hours when you are all alone in a bad area of town with felony suspects, for units from other nearby divisions to come to my aid.

I could write a novel on all the horrific incidents that happened to me, but that is not the purpose of this book.

The point of this book is to implore individuals and corporations to get their heads out of the sand; to see that not much has changed, at least not in LA, in the last twenty-five years. This is why I spend my time speaking on substance use disorders, mental health issues, and well-being strategies and writing this book in the hopes of reaching someone, like you, who needs backup.

Consider me your backup.

Between 1997 and 2000, I went through an incredible amount of stress, anxiety, and depression because of the disciplinary procedures the LAPD put me through. Those years were the darkest years of my life. It was so incomprehensible that I had to go on a leave of absence.

During this leave, I used up all of my overtime, sick, vacation, and whatever else time off I had to support my son and me. I decided that I could no longer continue living with all of the trauma, depression, stress, and anxiety, dealing with everything. I was a single, divorced mom.

I had to be a role model for my son.

I had to be strong.

I had to *step up and take action.*

In February of 2000, I walked away from a career that I loved.

It was devastating.

I knew that I was a strong, independent, educated, and determined woman and that I could do anything I put my mind to.

But we all have a breaking point.

During those three years, I broke into a million pieces like a shattered mirror, reflecting only distortions and jagged edges. It took some time to put myself back together.

I sought help from mental health professionals to deal with the trauma, depression, anxiety, and stress I endured. I found other survivors who had gone through the same or similar situations as I had fought my way through. They became my support network.

I continued my education and obtained my BS degree in Business Management. I took seminars on how to start a business.

Subsequently, I became a certified AFAA instructor and started teaching group exercise classes to stay physically fit. Getting into the fitness industry and teaching was one of the best decisions I ever made. Being around healthy, positive fitness professionals was a blessing. Once I had my physical body back into a positive mindset, everything else seemed to fall into place. My mindset continued to move in a forward, positive direction, and I became stronger emotionally, intellectually, and spiritually.

I obtained my Private Investigator license and started my PI firm. I went to law school and obtained my JD. Neither one of these goals was an easy accomplishment. No one in my immediate family graduated from high school or owned a business. I had no role models or mentors in my family. I had to be the role model and be the first to succeed on so many levels.

It took that amount of time and a different focus of desperation, but I realized that healing was more important than upholding my truth and defending my reputation. It had, indeed, taken all costs—and yet remained incomplete. I closed the chapter of my life with the LAPD, and I moved on. I found and used all of the tools and resources to help me become a resilient person again.

Steps 5 and 6 are the "action" phase of The ABELLA Model. If you have done the foundational work of the first four steps and surfaced the mental and emotional patterns that have been holding you back so you can heal, the action you take *now* can transform your life. Or your organization's culture and wellness.

Step 5: Link and Leverage

"The greatest leverage you can create for yourself is the pain that comes from inside, not outside."—Tony Robbins.

Link and Leverage represent the *initiation of action* by strategically connecting resources—internal strengths, external supports, and organizational tools—and deploying them to build resilience. This step transforms awareness and learning into tangible strategies: implementing self-care practices, strengthening professional networks, and advocating for trauma-informed policies. Without leveraging, knowledge remains theoretical; action here creates the scaffolding for sustainable change.

Step 6: Apply Action

"If you can't fly, then run. If you can't run, then walk. If you can't walk, then crawl, but whatever you do, you have to keep moving forward."—Martin Luther King, Jr.

Apply Action embodies *sustained, purposeful action*— consistently applying trauma-informed strategies to achieve balance, purpose, and growth. This step moves beyond temporary fixes to embed resilience into daily practice, fostering leadership and cultural transformation. It turns intention into identity, where individuals become role models and organizations evolve toward empathy-driven effectiveness.

You cannot sustain action without first linking to resources. Leveraging builds the support system—tools, networks, policies—that will make sustained action possible. Leveraging provides the "how," and then Apply Action provides the "why." Without having the resources, support, or tools to help you, taking action may backfire and set you up for failure.

I know how hard it is to start all over. I was 41 years old and I had no money when I left the LAPD and started my new life and business. I had to think strategically and figure it out. I had to take action and continue to move forward.

The lesson I learned from my 20 years in the LAPD is that everyone is replaceable. I gave my entire life to the department, and it cast me away like a ship out to sea without a care. I put the LAPD before my family and even my own sanity. All along, they treated me like I was disposable. My family and my well-being will always come before any career or business.

I see this all the time as a fitness instructor and health and wellness coach. Many people want to lose weight. They try every diet under the sun and may go to support groups, but they don't exercise. Or maybe they exercise, but eat everything they see. In order to be fit and healthy, there are several factors that must be considered. You must take your MEDS. You must be willing to (1) change your **m**indset, (2) have an **e**stablished exercise routine, (3) eat a healthy and nutritious **d**iet, and (4) get sufficient **s**leep.

If you have any medical issues, there could be other contributing factors that you must take into consideration. You must really want to lose weight, commit to what needs to be done, and be accountable, which is why many people hire a personal trainer or fitness and/or health and wellness coach to help them stay on track and as an accountability partner. Once you have all the pieces of the puzzle, you can start putting them in the correct slots, and the "big picture" will appear!

I know that this is a lot to digest, learn, and remember, especially if you are one who is dealing with any of these types of issues. Sometimes you feel frozen and figure, "If I just close my eyes, it will all go away." Or you can get pulled right back into guilt and shame for the place where you are as a result of the events that occurred in your life, and not having had the support to put those in their proper place and begin to heal.

We all know that is not reality. You don't have to do this alone. Having an accountability partner by itself is a valuable resource to help you get on track. As a coach and consultant, I can help you achieve each of these steps in order so that this time, all the work you invest serves to improve your personal and professional development. For leaders of businesses and organizations, as a trainer, facilitator, and public speaker, I can help you develop trauma-informed policies and procedures and train your staff.

If you fail to link and leverage trauma-informed resources and support, you will risk falling back or remaining stuck in old patterns, missing the chance to achieve meaningful, lasting transformation.

Action is the engine of transformation: It's what turns all the ideas, intentions, and dreams we hold into tangible results.

Whether you're writing a book, growing a business, or stepping into your role as a powerful messenger, action is what sets you apart from those who only talk or plan.

When you take action, you build momentum, gather real-world feedback, and discover what works, allowing you to adjust, improve, and keep moving forward. Without action, even the best ideas remain unrealized, and opportunities slip away. We ran out of time. We miss out on our best lives, with the results of our powerful ideas and inspiration unrealized.

When we rush into action without first doing the inner work, such as going through all of the steps of The ABELLA Model in order, we waste energy on misaligned goals and risk setbacks that erode our confidence and self-trust. We fall back too readily into old patterns, triggered by thoughts, feelings, experiences, and reactions we have long forgotten about.

Have you ever noticed this happening to you?

Acting without clarity often leads to frustration and stalled progress, making it harder to believe in ourselves. Ironically, slowing down to reflect and align our intentions, do the deep emotional work to see ourselves and our contexts fully, and reflect on the role that our own personal agency can play to shift our trajectory—that is what so many people want to skip in order to get out of pain faster. That painstaking process *is* the work that is key to the faster, more meaningful results—ensuring that every step we take is purposeful and truly transformative.

The core insight behind Step 5, Link and Leverage, and Step 6, Apply Action, is that true transformation isn't about doing *more*—it's about doing what matters most, with intention—

and from a place of inner alignment rather than reactivity.

It took me a while to learn how my reactivity could send me down the wrong path. Without awareness of what was triggering me, I would respond in ways that got me the opposite results I had hoped for.

When you link to the right resources and take purposeful action, you move forward with clarity, resilience, and impact, rather than simply staying busy (masking your avoidance or blame) or overwhelmed (not seeing the proper actions to take, so you try all of them) or racing on the hamster wheel to nowhere.

My role as your coach, consultant, or facilitator is to walk beside you as your accountability partner, helping you stay rooted in your values and focused on what truly moves you and/or your organization forward. Together, we'll ensure every step you take is both grounded and meaningful, so you can create lasting change where it matters most.

As you can see, to transform, there are certain steps you must take. If you are dealing with these mental health issues, you have to "face it to fix it," which is amplifying awareness. Next, you have to "drop the drama and ditch the blame," which is moving beyond blame and stopping the excuses. Then you must examine and evaluate your mental, emotional, and physical well-being, identify warning signs, and confront inaction. Once you have absorbed the knowledge about trauma and resilience, you must listen and learn about it from experts, peers, and your own experiences. Next, you will link and leverage by connecting resources and strategically deploying them. You will end by applying action and trauma-informed strategies to achieve balance and purpose.

If you're ready to turn insight into real, lasting change—whether for yourself or your organization—the most powerful next step is to bring in expert support. In the next chapter, I'll show you how working with me as your coach or consultant can accelerate your growth and create a trauma-informed culture where everyone thrives.

To deepen your understanding and apply the insights from this chapter, I invite you to visit **www.LitaAbella.com** and use the interactive journal with seven guided questions—designed to help you reflect, plan, and take action on your journey toward resilience and well-being.

NEXT STEPS

You've walked through the steps of The ABELLA Model and now hold the keys to personal and organizational renewal in your hands. But as you know, information alone doesn't change lives—what matters is what you do next.

I've been where you are, feeling stuck, overwhelmed, or uncertain about how to turn insight into action. I know how tempting it is to stay in the comfort zone, to keep running on that hamster wheel of blame and avoidance, convincing yourself that nothing will change. I've been there, too—playing it safe, pointing fingers, and waiting until it almost felt too late.

But here's the truth: transformation is possible, and it starts with a choice. You have three paths ahead of you.

Option 1: Change Nothing. Stay Where You Are

You can keep doing what you've always done, hoping for a different result. The comfort zone feels safe, but it's also where dreams go to fade. If you're a leader, CEO, or someone with influence in your business or organization, remember: Your choices ripple out to your team, your family, and your community. When you change nothing, nothing changes—and the world misses out on the impact only you can make.

Option 2: Do It Yourself

Maybe you're determined to try this on your own. I respect that. It's brave. But I also know how lonely and exhausting it can be—how your own mind can become your toughest critic, whispering doubts and holding you back. You might make progress, but it's slow, and it's easy to lose hope. If, after a month or two, you're still stuck or struggling, please don't keep suffering alone. If information alone were enough to transform you, it's likely you could have done that by now.

Option 3: Let's Talk—I Can Help

I'm not just offering coaching, consulting, facilitating, and training; I'm offering a hand to hold and a heart that genuinely understands. As a board-certified coach, licensed private investigator, and former law enforcement officer, I know how to listen actively and ask powerful questions. As an entrepreneur, I know how important it is to have a reputable brand, a profitable business, and satisfied customers. I also know how important it is to have happy and healthy staff who are proud to work for an organization.

I've walked through trauma, burnout, and reinvented myself. I know how hard it is to ask for help and worry about the stigma around it. I also know how powerful it is to have someone truly listen, without judgment, with empathy, and with proven experience to guide you forward.

I've seen individual clients through this process and watched it transform their lives, and you can do the same.

I had a coaching client who suffered from a traumatic childhood, dealing with verbal and physical abuse from her mother. She had no role models in her family and was a teenage mother herself. I didn't discover this information until several sessions with her because she had never talked with anyone about her pain and trauma.

She now had a 16-year-old son, who was only 15 years younger than her. She wanted to be a good mom to her son, but it was difficult because she needed to deal with her own issues and challenges. She desperately needed help from a mental health professional to deal with all of the trauma in her life. I was finally able to talk her into making an appointment with a licensed mental health professional. Once she started receiving treatment from her therapist, it was a life-changing experience for her. She is now in a much better place with herself and her son. However, it took the coaching sessions from me to show her what she needed to move forward in her life.

All it takes is one conversation—one honest, open, and compassionate talk—to change everything. Having an accountability partner makes it so much more manageable to implement change.

Please don't wait. Reach out. Let's start with a free 30-minute session to explore how I can support your journey. Whether you're an individual ready for change, or a leader or CEO wanting to build a trauma-informed, resilient organization.

For instance, I can provide engaging and informative presentations, help develop trauma-informed policies, and train your staff on trauma-informed practices. I'm here for you.

Contact me at **Lita@LitaAbella.com** or visit www.LitaAbella. com. Thank you for reading my book and for taking the first step toward the future you deserve.

THE FINAL CHAPTER

I have had a very interesting personal life, as well as my professional 45-year career, with a lot of ups and downs. I'm not going to say that my life at the age of 66 is perfect because it is not, but seeking perfection, I have found, exacerbates an already untenable situation.

There were a lot of mistakes I made throughout my life, as well as many outstanding accomplishments. I'm still learning about life at this senior age!

My parents were not wealthy, but they owned the house I grew up in—in Hollywood. My mother was a mixed-race, Caucasian and African-American, from New Orleans, LA. My father was Filipino, born and raised in Ilocos Sur, a province in the Philippines. He spoke Ilocano and broken English, which has a lot of the Spanish language, which made it easy for me to pick up the Spanish language. I have a younger brother, who is four years my junior. I had an older half-brother and half-sister, who were half-Filipino and half-Mexican.

Neither of my parents graduated from high school. All they wanted for my brother and me was to graduate from high school. Our parents raised us to be respectful, decent people. Other than the beatings by my mom, we had a pretty normal life. We never had an encounter with the police, and the police were never called to our house.

You can imagine what a shock it was for me to get married and become a domestic violence victim, join the LAPD, see nothing but the unspeakable scenes, and go through three divorces by the age of 32.

In the process, I learned compassion. I also found my passion: Speaking out, speaking up, and raising awareness of trauma-informed support for helping professionals and those who experience PTSD, vicarious trauma, compassion fatigue, and burnout in disproportionate shares. I am not a mental health professional. However, I understand these issues because I have *experienced* them myself and have worked with others (the public, clients, and professionals) who have experienced them in my 45-year career.

I now speak on stages across the country, advocating and educating professionals in high-stress professions on the importance of having trauma-informed practices.

During my last six years at the State Bar of California, I worked in the Office of Professional Competence, Lawyer Assistance Program, and gave over 400 educational MCLE presentations to attorneys and legal professionals on substance use disorders, mental health issues, and wellness strategies. That is how great the need was and still is.

In doing so, I saw the need for professionals in the "helping others" industry to be educated on these types of topics. I conducted research and discovered that most professionals do not have sufficient training on mental health issues.

For example, most attorneys in the US are only required to obtain one to two hours of mental health/substance abuse training every two to three years. In California, law enforcement officers receive eight hours of training in the academy, and when they become field training officers, they receive four hours of crisis intervention behavioral health training.

Coaches are not regulated significantly in the sense of being required to be licensed, trained, or certified. The International Coaching Federation (ICF), a global organization that oversees credentialing for coaches, encourages coaches to continually develop their skills and knowledge, which can include seeking additional training in areas such as mental health. However, the formal credentialing process doesn't require a specific number of mental health-related training hours.

I believe knowledge is power, and I strongly advocate for professionals to be educated in their area of expertise. I am an ICF Associate Certified Coach, Board Certified Coach with the Center for Credentialing and Education, and Wellcoaches Certified Health and Well-Being Coach.

As you can see, many individuals who work in sensitive fields do not receive sufficient training in the area of mental health. The goal of my book is to help others dealing with these issues by implementing The ABELLA Model so that those affected can get help and workplaces and organizations can implement trauma-informed practices that will help the individual, the customers they serve, and the organization.

I also hope that those industries that are regulated by the government or a regulatory agency will require their licensees or certified professionals to receive sufficient training on these types of issues so that individuals are better informed and trained and can better serve the public. I continue to educate myself on these important issues and advocate for training in all the industries that could be affected.

I hope that if you are dealing with these issues, you reach out, get help, seek support, and educate yourself.

I am here if you would like to talk, provide feedback, suggestions, or comments. Please contact me at **Lita@LitaAbella.com**.

ABOUT THE AUTHOR

Lita Abella holds a JD degree from Western State University College of Law and has experience as a law clerk for prosecutorial agencies. This legal foundation equips her with a deep understanding of conflict resolution and the complexities of the legal field.

As the founder of Lita Abella Coaching, Consulting & Mediation Services, she specializes in coaching and consulting, guiding individuals and organizations to unlock their full potential. As a mediator, she is dedicated to facilitating effective communication and helping parties reach amicable resolutions. Her approach to mediation is client-centered, focusing on empathy, neutrality, and facilitating open dialogue to achieve mutually beneficial outcomes.

With over a decade of service at the State Bar of California in various investigative and leadership roles, Lita has demonstrated exceptional problem-solving skills, a strong commitment to fairness, and tireless advocacy for workers' rights. Her experience in the Office of Chief Trial Counsel, where she assisted in investigating and prosecuting attorney misconduct, provides her with insights into the pressures that legal professionals face, including the risks of disciplinary actions and malpractice lawsuits.

Lita is a seasoned public speaker, delivering educational presentations to attorneys on critical topics such as substance use disorders, mental health, and work-life balance. Her diverse background with the LAPD highlights her resilience, adaptability, and leadership under pressure. She understands the emotional toll that high-stress careers can take, particularly regarding post-traumatic stress, vicarious trauma, and compassion fatigue.

Lita is a licensed private investigator and an entrepreneur with 25 years of experience. Her long-standing involvement in the fitness, health, and wellness industry underscores her commitment to personal well-being and holistic growth. Lastly, she is a professor of business law and paralegal studies, sharing her expertise with the next generation of legal professionals.

ACKNOWLEDGMENTS

I am deeply grateful to all the individuals I have had the privilege to work with—whether leading or following your lead—your trust and collaboration have been invaluable.

To my family, friends, and close colleagues, thank you for your unwavering faith, guidance, and steadfast support throughout this journey; your encouragement has sustained me more than words can express.

"No one who achieves success does so without acknowledging the help of others. The wise and confident acknowledge this help with gratitude."—Alfred North Whitehead.

BEFORE YOU GO...

Assess Your Well-Being

PTSD, Vicarious Trauma, Compassion Fatigue, and Burnout Self-Assessments are four separate screening tools to determine if you **may** be experiencing the signs and symptoms of these issues. It is not a diagnosis, but it can start a conversation between you and someone qualified to diagnose and treat. It's short and insightful, and it's free. You'll find it at **www.LitaAbella.com**.

Want The **ABELLA** Model Cheat Sheet?

Would you like a **cheat sheet** of The ABELLA Model to help remind you of the six steps you'll need to take to go from overwhelmed and stuck to empowered and resilient? Send an email to Lita@LitaAbella.com and put 'SEND ME THE CHEAT SHEET' in the subject line.

The **ABELLA** Model: Trauma-Informed Coaching Program

The ABELLA Model is the prequel to my signature coaching program, The ABELLA Model: Trauma-Informed Coaching

Program, which takes people from overwhelmed and stuck to empowered and resilient.

To experience true and lasting healing, growth, and professional fulfillment, The ABELLA Model: Trauma-Informed Coaching Program prepares your mind to accomplish clarity, confidence, and sustainable transformation—whether you're healing from trauma, supporting others through their struggles, or leading teams in high-stress environments.

Let me help you or your organization move beyond survival and into a future defined by strength, purpose, and well-being by providing one-on-one coaching, group coaching, or team coaching services. For more information about how you can participate in the program, visit **www.LitaAbella.com**.

The ABELLA Model: Trauma-Informed Training for Professionals

The ABELLA Model: Trauma-Informed Training for Professionals Program takes individuals and teams from overwhelmed and reactive to empowered and resilient, with content and strategies specifically tailored to your industry—whether legal, healthcare, public service, education, or beyond. Training is delivered in a customized one-day workshop.

This training program equips professionals with the clarity, confidence, and practical tools needed to navigate trauma, support clients and colleagues, and foster a culture of sustainable transformation. They come to experience true and lasting well-being, effectiveness, and organizational strength. The training provides trauma-informed practices with real-world application for your particular industry.

Empower your team to move beyond survival; create a workplace defined by purpose, compassion, and resilience, uniquely designed for the challenges of your field.

If this book resonated with you, I would truly appreciate you taking a moment to share a review. You may leave your review on the following platforms:

Amazon

Google Business Profile

Goodreads

For more information about how you can participate in the program, visit **www.LitaAbella.com**.

Thank you for your interest in

THE ABELLA MODEL

By Lita E. Abella, JD, BCC, ACC

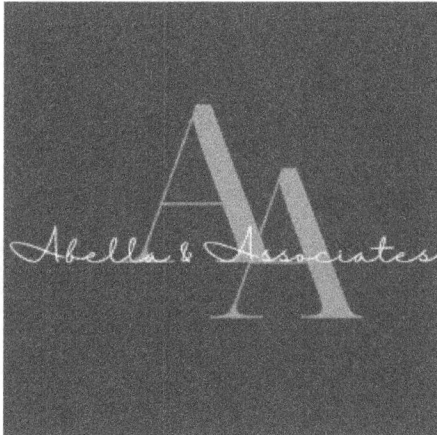

Published by:
Abella and Associates Group LLC

www.ingramcontent.com/pod-product-compliance
Lightning Source LLC
Chambersburg PA
CBHW060400050426
42449CB00009B/1834